THE BEANS DIET

LOSE WEIGHT THE EASIEST AND HEALTHY WAY

BY

ADELE

WORCESTER

All rights reserved. No part of this publication may be reproduced, distributed, or transmitted in any form or by any means, including photocopying, recording, or other electronic or mechanical methods, without the prior written permission of the publisher, except in the case of brief quotations embodied in critical reviews and certain other noncommercial uses permitted by copyright law.

Copyright © Adele Worcester, 2024

Disclaimer:The information provided in this book, "The Beans Diet: Lose Weight the Easiest and Healthy Way," is intended for educational and informational purposes only. The content presented in this book is not intended to serve as a substitute for professional medical advice, diagnosis, or treatment. Always seek the advice of your physician or other qualified healthcare provider with any questions you may have regarding a medical condition or dietary regimen.The author and publisher of this book are not liable for any adverse effects or consequences resulting from the use or misuse of the information presented herein. Readers are encouraged to consult with a qualified health care professional before making any changes to their diet, exercise routine, or lifestyle based on the information provided in this book.Individual results may vary, and the success of any weight loss or dietary program depends on various factors, including but not limited to an individual's overall health, medical history, genetics, and adherence to the program. The author and publisher make no guarantees or warranties regarding the accuracy, completeness, or suitability of the information provided in this book for any particular purpose.Readers are responsible for their own health and well-being and should use their discretion when implementing any recommendations or suggestions outlined in this book. Any reliance on the information provided in this book is done at the reader's own risk.By reading this book, you acknowledge and agree to the terms of this disclaimer. If you do not agree with these terms, you should not use the information provided in this book.

TABLE OF CONTENTS

Chapter 1
Introduction to the Beans Diet

Chapter 2
Getting Started with the Beans Diet

Chapter 3
Exploring Different Varieties of Beans

Chapter 4
Incorporating Beans into Your Favourite Recipes

Chapter 5
The Science Behind the Beans Diet

Chapter 6
Tips for Success on the Beans Diet

Chapter 7
Sustainable Lifestyle Changes for Long-Term Success

Chapter 8
Maintaining Success and Embracing a Lifetime of Health

Chapter 9
Conclusion

Chapter 1

Introduction to the Beans Diet

Welcome to "The Beans Diet: Lose Weight the Easiest and Healthy Way"!

In a world inundated with fad diets and quick-fix solutions, the Beans Diet offers a refreshing and sustainable approach to weight loss and overall health.The Beans Diet is not just another trendy diet plan; it is a lifestyle change rooted in centuries-old culinary traditions and backed by modern nutritional science. Beans, legumes that encompass a wide variety of plant species, have been a staple food in cultures around the globe for millennia. From lentils to chickpeas, black beans to kidney beans, these humble legumes pack a powerful nutritional punch that forms the cornerstone of the Beans Diet.At the heart of the Beans Diet lies the recognition of beans as a nutritional powerhouse. Rich in protein, fiber, vitamins, minerals, and antioxidants, beans offer a myriad of health benefits that support weight loss and overall well-being. Unlike many processed and refined foods that dominate modern diets, beans are a natural and whole food source that nourishes the body while promoting satiety and sustained energy levels.One of the key advantages of the Beans Diet is its simplicity. Gone are the days of counting calories or meticulously measuring portion sizes. With the Beans Diet, you can enjoy a diverse array of delicious and satisfying meals while effortlessly managing your weight. Whether you're a busy professional, a parent juggling multiple responsibilities, or someone simply looking for a convenient and nutritious way to eat, the Beans Diet offers a practical solution that fits seamlessly into any lifestyle.Moreover, the Beans Diet is not just about shedding excess pounds; it's about fostering a holistic approach to health. By incorporating beans into your daily meals, you're not only fueling your body with essential nutrients but also reducing your risk of chronic diseases such as heart disease, diabetes, and certain cancers. The Beans Diet empowers you to take control of your health and make informed choices that prioritise long-term wellness.In this book, we will delve deeper into the science behind the Beans Diet, explore the various types of beans and their nutritional profiles, provide practical tips for success, and offer a wealth of delicious recipes to inspire your culinary creativity.

Whether you're embarking on your weight loss journey or simply seeking to improve your health, "The Beans Diet" is your comprehensive guide to achieving your goals the easiest and healthiest way possible.

Understanding the Benefits of Beans

Beans, often referred to as legumes, are a diverse group of plant foods that have been consumed by humans for thousands of years. From chickpeas to black beans, lentils to kidney beans, these nutrient-dense legumes offer a wide range of health benefits that make them a valuable addition to any diet.One of the most notable benefits of beans is their high nutritional content. They are an excellent source of plant-based protein, making them an ideal option for vegetarians and vegans looking to meet their protein needs. In addition to protein, beans are rich in complex carbohydrates, fiber, vitamins, and minerals. This nutrient profile not only provides sustained energy but also supports overall health and well-being.Fiber is a particularly important component of beans that contributes to their numerous health benefits. Soluble fiber, found in abundance in beans, helps to lower cholesterol levels, stabilise blood sugar levels, and promote a healthy digestive system. Insoluble fiber adds bulk to the stool, aiding in regularity and preventing constipation. By incorporating beans into your diet, you can significantly improve your digestive health and reduce your risk of developing chronic conditions such as heart disease, diabetes, and colon cancer.Another key benefit of beans is their low glycemic index (GI), which means they cause a gradual and steady rise in blood sugar levels. This makes them an excellent choice for individuals with diabetes or those looking to manage their blood sugar levels more effectively. By replacing high-GI foods with beans, you can help regulate your blood sugar levels and reduce your risk of insulin resistance and type 2 diabetes.Beans are also rich in antioxidants, compounds that help protect the body against oxidative stress and inflammation. Antioxidants play a crucial role in preventing chronic diseases and promoting overall health. By consuming beans regularly, you can boost your antioxidant intake and support your body's natural defence mechanisms.Additionally, beans are an affordable and versatile food option that can be incorporated into a wide variety of dishes. From soups and stews to salads and dips, the culinary possibilities are endless. Whether you're looking to add more plant-based foods to your diet, improve your overall health, or manage your weight, beans offer a convenient and nutritious solution.In summary, the benefits of beans are numerous and far-reaching. From their high nutritional content to their role in promoting digestive health and managing blood sugar levels, beans are a valuable addition to any diet. By incorporating beans into your meals regularly, you can reap the many health benefits they have to offer and take a significant step towards improving your overall well-being.

Why Beans Are Essential for Weight Loss

When it comes to weight loss, beans emerge as an essential and invaluable food group due to their unique nutritional composition and various properties that support weight management. Incorporating beans into your diet can significantly contribute to your weight loss journey in several ways.First and foremost, beans are exceptionally high in dietary fiber, which plays a crucial role in weight loss and weight management. Fiber-rich foods like beans promote feelings of fullness and satiety, which can help control appetite and reduce overall calorie intake. Additionally, fiber slows down the digestion process, leading to a more gradual release of glucose into the bloodstream and preventing rapid spikes in blood sugar levels. This steady release of energy helps maintain stable energy levels throughout the day and reduces the likelihood of experiencing energy crashes and subsequent overeating.Moreover, the fiber content in beans also aids in promoting digestive health. A healthy digestive system is essential for efficient nutrient absorption and waste elimination, both of which are important factors in supporting weight loss efforts. By keeping the digestive system functioning optimally, beans help ensure that the body is able to extract and utilise nutrients from food more effectively, thereby supporting overall metabolic function and weight management.In addition to their fiber content, beans are also an excellent source of plant-based protein. Protein is known to be highly satiating and can help increase feelings of fullness and reduce appetite, leading to decreased calorie consumption. Unlike many animal protein sources, beans are low in fat and cholesterol, making them a healthier option for individuals looking to lose weight while still meeting their protein in needs.Furthermore, beans are a nutrient-dense food, meaning they provide a significant amount of vitamins, minerals, and antioxidants relative to their calorie content. This makes them an ideal food choice for those looking to lose weight without sacrificing essential nutrients and overall health. By incorporating beans into your meals, you can ensure that you are getting a wide range of essential nutrients that support overall well-being while simultaneously managing your weight. Beans are incredibly versatile and can be incorporated into a variety of dishes, making them a convenient and accessible food option for individuals looking to lose weight. Whether added to soups, salads, stews, or stir-fries, beans can enhance the nutritional value and satiety of meals without significantly increasing calorie intake.In conclusion, beans are essential for weight loss due to their high fiber and protein content, nutrient density, and versatility. By incorporating beans into your diet, you can support satiety, promote digestive health, and ensure that you are getting essential nutrients while working towards your weight loss goals

Chapter 2

Getting Started with the Beans Diet

Congratulations on taking the first step towards a healthier lifestyle by choosing to embark on the Beans Diet journey! In this chapter, we will guide you through the essential steps to get started with the Beans Diet, including setting your weight loss goals, preparing your kitchen and pantry, and understanding the fundamental principles of this dietary approach.Setting Your Weight Loss Goals:Before diving into any diet or weight loss program, it's crucial to establish clear and realistic goals. Take some time to reflect on why you want to lose weight and what specific outcomes you hope to achieve through the Beans Diet. Are you looking to improve your overall health, boost your energy levels, or fit into your favourite pair of jeans? By setting specific, measurable, achievable, relevant, and time-bound (SMART) goals, you can create a roadmap for success and stay motivated throughout your journey.When setting your weight loss goals, it's essential to be realistic and avoid setting overly ambitious targets that may be difficult to attain. Aim for gradual, sustainable weight loss of 1-2 pounds per week, as this is considered a safe and healthy rate of weight loss. Remember that every individual is unique, and your weight loss journey may differ from others, so focus on progress rather than perfection.

Preparing Your Kitchen and Pantry

Creating a supportive environment in your kitchen and pantry is essential for successfully following the Beans Diet. Start by conducting a thorough inventory of your current food supplies and identifying any items that may not align with the Beans Diet principles, such as processed foods, sugary snacks, and refined carbohydrates. Consider donating or discarding these items to eliminate temptation and make room for nutrient-dense foods that support your weight loss goals.Next, stock up on a variety of beans and legumes to incorporate into your meals and snacks. Choose from a wide range of options, including black beans, chickpeas, lentils, kidney beans, and more, to keep your meals exciting and diverse. Opt for both canned and dried beans, keeping in mind that canned beans offer convenience and quick preparation, while dried beans can be cost-effective and provide more control over seasoning and sodium content.In addition to beans, ensure that your kitchen is equipped with essential tools and equipment for preparing bean-based meals, such as a stockpot, saucepan, slow cooker, and blender. Invest in high-quality cooking oils, herbs, and spices to add flavour to your dishes without relying on excessive salt or unhealthy fats.

Understanding the Fundamental Principles of the Beans Diet

At its core, the Beans Diet is a plant-based dietary approach that emphasises the consumption of beans and legumes as a primary source of protein, fiber, vitamins, and minerals. Unlike restrictive fad diets that focus on calorie counting or eliminating entire food groups, the Beans Diet encourages a balanced and sustainable approach to eating that prioritises whole, nutrient-dense foods.One of the key principles of the Beans Diet is portion control. While beans are nutritious and filling, it's important to practise portion control to avoid overeating and consuming excess calories. A typical serving size of cooked beans is about half a cup, which provides approximately 7-10 grams of protein and 6-8 grams of fiber, depending on the variety.Another fundamental principle of the Beans Diet is meal planning and preparation. By planning your meals ahead of time and preparing nutritious bean-based dishes in advance, you can avoid last-minute temptations to indulge in unhealthy foods and ensure that you have healthy options readily available when hunger strikes. Experiment with different recipes and meal combinations to keep your meals exciting and enjoyable.In addition to incorporating beans into your meals, the Beans Diet encourages the consumption of a variety of other plant-based foods, including fruits, vegetables, whole grains, nuts, and seeds. These foods provide essential nutrients and antioxidants that support overall health and well-being while complementing the nutritional benefits of beans.

Chapter 3

Types of Beans and Their Nutritional Value

In chapter 2, we discussed the fundamental principles of the Beans Diet and how to get started with incorporating beans into your diet. Now, let's delve deeper into the world of beans by exploring the various types of beans available and their nutritional value. Understanding the different varieties of beans and their unique nutritional profiles will empower you to make informed choices and create delicious, nutrient-dense meals that support your weight loss goals.

Types of Beans

Beans come in a wide array of shapes, sizes, and colours, each with its own distinct flavour and texture. From creamy black beans to nutty chickpeas, there's a bean variety to suit every palate and culinary preference. Let's take a closer look at some of the most popular types of beans and their characteristics:

Black Beans:Black beans, also known as turtle beans, are small, shiny, and jet-black in color.They have a creamy texture and a slightly sweet, earthy flavor.Black beans are a rich source of protein, fiber, folate, iron, and antioxidants.They are commonly used in Latin American and Caribbean cuisines, including soups, stews, and rice dishes.

Kidney Beans:Kidney beans are large, kidney-shaped beans that come in various colours, including red, white, and speckled.They have a hearty texture and a mild, slightly sweet flavor.Kidney beans are high in protein, fiber, folate, manganese, and potassium.They are commonly used in chilli, salads, and bean-based dips like hummus.

Chickpeas (Garbanzo Beans):Chickpeas are round, beige-coloured beans with a nutty flavour and firm texture.They are rich in protein, fiber, folate, iron, and magnesium.Chickpeas are a staple ingredient in Mediterranean and Middle Eastern cuisines, used in dishes such as hummus, falafel, and salads.

Lentils:Lentils are small, lens-shaped legumes that come in various colours, including green, red, brown, and black.They have a mild, earthy flavour and a soft texture when cooked.Lentils are an excellent source of protein, fiber, folate, iron, and potassium.They are versatile and can be used in a wide range of dishes, including soups, stews, salads, and curries.

Navy Beans:Navy beans, also known as haricot beans, are small, oval-shaped beans with a creamy white color.They have a mild flavour and a smooth, creamy texture when cooked.Navy beans are high in protein, fiber, folate, manganese, and phosphorus.They are commonly used in baked beans, soups, and casseroles.

Nutritional Value of Beans

Beans are renowned for their exceptional nutritional value and health benefits. They are a rich source of plant-based protein, making them an excellent alternative to meat for vegetarians and vegans. In addition to protein, beans are packed with dietary fiber, vitamins, minerals, and antioxidants that contribute to overall health and well-being.

Let's explore the nutritional composition of beans in more detail

Protein:Beans are a valuable source of plant-based protein, containing approximately 15-20 grams of protein per cooked cup, depending on the variety.Protein is essential for building and repairing tissues, supporting muscle growth and maintenance, and regulating various physiological processes in the body.

Fiber:Beans are high in dietary fiber, with approximately 12-15 grams of fiber per cooked cup, depending on the variety.Fiber plays a crucial role in digestive health, promoting regular bowel movements, preventing constipation, and reducing the risk of colon cancer.Additionally, fiber helps control blood sugar levels, improve cholesterol levels, and promote satiety, which can aid in weight loss and weight management.

Vitamins:Beans are rich in various vitamins, including folate, vitamin B6, vitamin K, and vitamin C, depending on the variety.Folate is essential for DNA synthesis and cell division, making it particularly important during periods of rapid growth and development, such as pregnancy.Vitamin B6 plays a role in protein metabolism, red blood cell formation, and neurotransmitter synthesis, supporting overall health and well-being.

Minerals:Beans are a good source of several minerals, including iron, magnesium, potassium, and zinc, depending on the variety.Iron is essential for oxygen transport in the blood, energy production, and immune function.Magnesium plays a role in muscle and nerve function, blood sugar regulation, and bone health.Potassium helps regulate blood pressure, fluid balance, and muscle contractions.Zinc is involved in immune function, wound healing, and DNA synthesis.

Antioxidants:Beans contain various antioxidants, including flavonoids, phenolic compounds, and carotenoids, which help protect cells from oxidative damage caused by free radicals.Antioxidants have anti-inflammatory and anti-cancer properties, and they may help reduce the risk of chronic diseases, such as heart disease, diabetes, and certain cancers.

Incorporating Beans into Your Diet

Now that you have a better understanding of the different types of beans and their nutritional value, it's time to start incorporating them into your diet.

Here are some tips for incorporating beans into your meals and snacks:

Experiment with Different Varieties:Try experimenting with different types of beans to discover your favourites and add variety to your diet. Consider incorporating a variety of colours and textures, such as black beans, chickpeas, lentils, and kidney beans.

Use Beans as a Protein Source

Replace meat with beans as a protein source in your meals. Incorporate beans into soups, stews, salads, stir-fries, and casseroles to add protein and fiber to your dishes.

Make Bean-Based Dips and Spreads

Make homemade bean-based dips and spreads, such as hummus, black bean dip, or lentil pâté, to enjoy as a snack or appetizer with vegetables, whole grain crackers, or whole grain bread.

Add Beans to Salads and Grain Bowls

Add beans to salads and grain bowls to boost their protein and fiber content. Combine beans with leafy greens, whole grains, vegetables, nuts, seeds, and a flavorful dressing for a nutritious and satisfying meal.

Incorporate Beans into Breakfast

Add beans to your breakfast routine by incorporating them into omelettes, scrambles, breakfast burritos, or savoury oatmeal. You can also enjoy bean-based breakfast dishes, such as black bean and sweet potato hash or chickpea flour pancakes.

Snack on Roasted Chickpeas

Roast chickpeas in the oven with your favourite seasonings for a crunchy and satisfying snack. Enjoy roasted chickpeas on their own or sprinkle them over salads, soups, or yogurt for added flavour and texture.

Make Bean-Based Desserts

Get creative with bean-based desserts by using beans as a substitute for flour or butter in baked goods.

Chapter 4

Bean- based recipes

Each of the recipes makes four servings.
When cooking beans from scratch, measurements are equivalent to already cooked beans and not raw beans

NB: Each person's calorie requirements may be different and depends on many factors.

Black Bean Burger:

Ingredients:
1 can (15 oz) black beans, drained and rinsed
1/2 cup breadcrumbs
1/4 cup diced onions
1/4 cup diced bell peppers
1 teaspoon cumin
1 teaspoon chili powder
Salt and pepper to taste

Directions:

Mash black beans in a bowl.
Add breadcrumbs, onions, bell peppers, cumins, chili powder, salt, and pepper. Mix well.
Form into patties and cook on a skillet or grill until browned on both sides.
Calories (per serving, without bun): Approximately 150 calories

2.Mediterranean Chickpea Salad:

Ingredients:

1 can (15 oz) chickpeas, drained and rinsed
1 cup diced cucumber
1 cup diced tomatoes
1/4 cup diced red onion
2 tablespoons chopped fresh parsley
2 tablespoons olive oil
1 tablespoon lemon juice
Salt and pepper to taste

Directions:

In a large bowl, combine chickpeas, cucumber, tomatoes, red onion, and parsley. Drizzle with olive oil and lemon juice. Season with salt and pepper.
Toss to combine and serve chilled.
Calories (per serving): Approximately 200 calories.

3. Bean and Vegetable Stir-Fry:

Ingredients:

1 can (15 oz) mixed beans, drained and rinsed
2 cups mixed vegetables (bell peppers, broccoli, carrots, snap peas)
2 cloves garlic, minced
2 tablespoons soy sauce
1 tablespoon sesame oil
1 tablespoon olive oil
Salt and pepper to taste

Directions:

Heat olive oil in a large skillet or wok over medium-high heat.
Add minced garlic and stir-fry for 30 seconds.
Add mixed vegetables and stir-fry until crisp-tender.
Add mixed beans, soy sauce, and sesame oil. Stir-fry for another 2-3 minutes.
Season with salt and pepper to taste. Serve hot over cooked rice or noodles.
Calories (per serving): Approximately 180 calories.

4. Bean and Quinoa Stuffed Bell Peppers:

Ingredients:

4 bell peppers, halved and seeds removed
1 cup cooked quinoa
1 can (15 oz) black beans, drained and rinsed
1 cup diced tomatoes
1/2 cup diced onions
1/2 cup corn kernels
1 teaspoon cumin1 teaspoon chili powder
Salt and pepper to taste

Directions:

Preheat the oven to 375°F (190°C).
In a bowl, mix cooked quinoa, black beans, diced tomatoes, onions, corn, cumin, chilli powder, salt, and pepper.
Fill each bell pepper half with the quinoa-bean mixture.
Place stuffed peppers in a baking dish and cover with foil.

Bake for 25-30 minutes until peppers are tender.
Calories (per serving, 1 stuffed pepper half): Approximately 200 calories.

5. White Bean and Spinach Soup:

Ingredients:

1 can (15 oz) white beans, drained and rinsed
2 cups chopped spinach
1/2 cup diced onions
2 cloves garlic, minced
4 cups vegetable broth
1 tablespoon olive oil
Salt and pepper to taste

Directions:

Heat olive oil in a large pot over medium heat.
Add diced onions and minced garlic.

Sauté until softened.
Add vegetable broth and bring to a simmer.
Add white beans and chopped spinach. Simmer for 10-15 minutes.
Season with salt and pepper to taste. Serve hot.
Calories (per serving): Approximately 150 calories.

6. Black Bean and Corn Salsa:

Ingredients:1 can (15 oz) black beans, drained and rinsed
1 cup corn kernels (fresh or frozen, thawed)
1/2 cup diced tomatoes
1/4 cup diced red onion
2 tablespoons chopped fresh cilantro
2 tablespoons lime juice
1 tablespoon olive oil
Salt and pepper to taste

Directions:

In a bowl, combine black beans, corn, tomatoes, red onion, and cilantro.

In a separate small bowl, whisk together lime juice, olive oil, salt, and pepper.

Pour the dressing over the salsa mixture and toss to combine.

Serve chilled with tortilla chips or as a topping for tacos.

Calories (per serving, 1/2 cup): Approximately 120 calories.

7. Vegan Black Bean Soup:

Ingredients:2 cans (15 oz each) black beans, drained and rinsed

1 cup diced tomatoes

1/2 cup diced onions

2 cloves garlic, minced

4 cups vegetable broth

1 teaspoon cumin

1 teaspoon chili powder

Salt and pepper to taste

Directions:

In a large pot, sauté onions and garlic until softened.

Add diced tomatoes, black beans, vegetable broth, cumin, chili powder, salt, and pepper.

Bring to a boil, then reduce heat and simmer for 20-30 minutes.

Use an immersion blender to partially blend the soup until desired consistency is reached.

Serve hot with optional toppings like avocado, cilantro, or tortilla strips.

Calories (per serving): Approximately 180 calories.

8. Three Bean Salad:

Ingredients:

1 can (15 oz) kidney beans, drained and rinsed

1 can (15 oz) chickpeas, drained and rinsed

1 can (15 oz) black beans, drained and rinsed

1/2 cup diced red onion

1/2 cup diced bell peppers (any colour)
1/4 cup chopped fresh parsley
2 tablespoons olive oil
2 tablespoons apple cider vinegar
Salt and pepper to taste

Directions:

In a large bowl, combine kidney beans, chickpeas, black beans, red onion, bell peppers, and parsley.
In a small bowl, whisk together olive oil, apple cider vinegar, salt, and pepper.
Pour the dressing over the bean mixture and toss to combine.
Chill in the refrigerator for at least 30 minutes before serving to allow flavours to meld.
Serve chilled as a side dish or as a topping for salads.
Calories (per serving, 1/2 cup): Approximately 200 calories.

9. Vegetarian Bean Tacos:I

Ingredients:1 can (15 oz) black beans, drained and rinsed
1 cup diced tomatoes
1/2 cup diced onions
1/2 cup diced bell peppers
1 teaspoon cumin1 teaspoon chili powder
Salt and pepper to taste
8 small corn or whole wheat tortillas
Optional toppings: shredded lettuce, diced avocado, salsa, shredded cheese

Directions:

In a skillet, sauté onions and bell peppers until softened.
Add diced tomatoes, black beans, cumin, chili powder, salt, and pepper.
 Cook until heated through.
Warm tortillas in a separate skillet or microwave.
Fill tortillas with the bean mixture.
Add optional toppings if desired.
Serve warm.

Calories (per serving, 2 tacos): Approximately 250 calories.

10. Vegan Bean Chili:

Ingredients:

2 cans (15 oz each) kidney beans, drained and rinsed
1 can (15 oz) black beans, drained and rinsed
1 can (15 oz) diced tomatoes
1 cup diced onions
1 cup diced bell peppers
2 cloves garlic, minced
2 tablespoons chili powder
1 teaspoon cumin
1 teaspoon paprika
Salt and pepper to taste

Directions:

In a large pot, sauté onions and bell peppers until softened.

Add minced garlic and cook for another minute.

Add diced tomatoes, kidney beans, black beans, chili powder, cumin, paprika, salt, and pepper.

Bring to a boil, then reduce heat and simmer for 20-30 minutes.

Serve hot with optional toppings like diced avocado, chopped cilantro, or vegan cheese.

Calories (per serving): Approximately 220 calories.

11. Bean and Vegetable Quesadillas:

Ingredients:

1 can (15 oz) refried beans
1 cup diced bell peppers
1/2 cup diced onions
1 cup diced tomatoes
1 cup shredded cheese (cheddar or Mexican blend)
8 small whole wheat tortillas
Olive oil or cooking spray

Directions:

Heat a skillet over medium heat and lightly grease with olive oil or cooking spray.
Spread refried beans on one side of each tortilla.
Top half of each tortilla with bell peppers, onions, tomatoes, and shredded cheese.
Fold tortillas in half and cook in the skillet until golden brown on both sides.
Cut quesadillas into wedges and serve hot.
Serving Size: Makes approximately 4 servings (2 quesadillas per serving).
Calories (per serving): Approximately 300 calories.

12. Black Bean and Avocado Wrap:

Ingredients:

1 can (15 oz) black beans, drained and rinsed
1 ripe avocado, mashed
1/4 cup diced red onion

1/4 cup diced bell peppers
1/4 cup diced tomatoes
4 whole wheat wraps
Salt and pepper to taste

Directions:

In a bowl, mix black beans, mashed avocado, red onion, bell peppers, and tomatoes.
Season with salt and pepper.
Spread the mixture onto each whole wheat wrap.
Roll up the wraps tightly and cut in half.
Serve immediately or wrap in foil for later.
Serving Size: Makes approximately 4 servings.
Calories (per serving): Approximately 250 calories.

13. Bean and Corn Stuffed Bell Peppers:

Ingredients:

4 bell peppers, halved and seeds removed
1 can (15 oz) black beans, drained and rinsed
1 cup cooked quinoa
1 cup corn kernels (fresh or frozen, thawed)
1/2 cup diced tomatoes
1/4 cup diced onions
1 teaspoon cumin
1 teaspoon chili powder
Salt and pepper to taste

Directions:

Preheat oven to 375°F (190°C).
In a bowl, mix black beans, cooked quinoa, corn kernels, diced tomatoes, onions, cumin, chili powder, salt, and pepper.
Fill each bell pepper half with the bean and corn mixture.
Place stuffed peppers in a baking dish and cover with foil.
Bake for 25-30 minutes until peppers are tender.

Serving Size: Makes approximately 4 servings (1 stuffed pepper half per serving). Calories (per serving): Approximately 200 calories.

14. Bean and Rice Burrito Bowl:

Ingredients:

I can (15 oz) black beans, drained and rinsed
2 cups cooked brown rice
1 cup diced tomatoes
1/2 cup diced onions
1/2 cup diced bell peppers
1/4 cup chopped fresh cilantro
1 avocado, sliced
1 lime, cut into wedges
Salt and pepper to taste

Directions:

In a bowl, layer cooked brown rice, black beans, diced tomatoes, onions, bell peppers, and chopped cilantro.

Top with sliced avocado.

Season with salt and pepper.

Serve with lime wedges for squeezing over the bowl.

Serving Size: Makes approximately 4 servings.

Calories (per serving): Approximately 300 calories.

15. Bean and Spinach Stuffed Mushrooms:

Ingredients:

12 large mushrooms, stems removed
1 can (15 oz) white beans, drained and rinsed
1 cup chopped spinach
1/4 cup diced onions
2 cloves garlic, minced
1/4 cup grated Parmesan cheese (optional)
Salt and pepper to taste

Directions:

Preheat the oven to 375°F (190°C).

In a bowl, mash white beans with a fork.

Add chopped spinach, diced onions, minced garlic, Parmesan cheese (if using), salt, and pepper. Mix well.

Stuff each mushroom cap with the bean and spinach mixture.

Place stuffed mushrooms on a baking sheet and bake for 15-20 minutes until mushrooms are tender.

Serving Size: Makes approximately 4 servings (3 mushrooms per serving).

Calories (per serving): Approximately 150 calories.

16. Bean and Corn Quesadilla:

Ingredients:

1 can (15 oz) pinto beans, drained and rinsed

1 cup corn kernels (fresh or frozen, thawed)

1/2 cup diced tomatoes

1/4 cup diced onions

1 teaspoon cumin

1 teaspoon chilli powder
Salt and pepper to taste
4 small whole wheat tortillas
1 cup shredded cheese (cheddar or Mexican blend)
Olive oil or cooking spray

Directions:

In a skillet, combine pinto beans, corn kernels, diced tomatoes, onions, cumin, chilli powder, salt, and pepper.

Cook over medium heat until heated through.

Heat a separate skillet over medium heat and lightly grease with olive oil or cooking spray.

Place one tortilla in the skillet and sprinkle with shredded cheese.

Spoon the bean and corn mixture over half of the tortilla.

Fold the other half of the tortilla over the filling and press down gently.

Cook for 2-3 minutes on each side until golden brown and crispy.
Repeat with remaining tortillas and filling.
Cut quesadillas into wedges and serve hot.
Serving Size: Makes approximately 4 servings (1 quesadilla per serving).
Calories (per serving): Approximately 300 calories.

17. Bean and Veggie Skewers:

Ingredients:

1 can (15 oz) cannellini beans, drained and rinsed
1 zucchini, sliced
1 bell pepper, diced
1 red onion, cut into chunksCherry tomatoes
2 tablespoons olive oil
2 tablespoons balsamic vinegar
1 teaspoon Italian seasoning
Salt and pepper to taste

Directions:

Preheat grill or grill pan over medium heat.

Thread cannellini beans, zucchini slices, bell pepper chunks, red onion chunks, and cherry tomatoes onto skewers.

In a small bowl, whisk together olive oil, balsamic vinegar, Italian seasoning, salt, and pepper.

Brush the skewers with the olive oil mixture.

Grill the skewers for 8-10 minutes, turning occasionally, until vegetables are tender and slightly charred.

Serve hot as a main dish or side dish.

Serving Size: Makes approximately 4 servings.

Calories (per serving): Approximately 200 calories.

18. Bean and Corn Salad with Cilantro-Lime Dressing:

Ingredients:

1 can (15 oz) black beans, drained and rinsed

1 cup corn kernels (fresh or frozen, thawed)
1 cup diced tomatoes
1/2 cup diced red onion
1/4 cup chopped fresh cilantro
2 tablespoons lime juice
2 tablespoons olive oil
1 teaspoon honey or agave syrup (optional)
Salt and pepper to taste

Directions:

In a large bowl, combine black beans, corn, tomatoes, red onion, and cilantro.
In a small bowl, whisk together lime juice, olive oil, honey or agave syrup (if using), salt, and pepper.
Pour the dressing over the bean mixture and toss to coat.
Serve chilled as a side dish or topping for tacos.Serving Size: Makes approximately 4 servings (1/2 cup per serving).Calories (per serving): Approximately 150 calories.

19. Bean and Rice Stuffed Peppers:

Ingredients:

4 bell peppers, halved and seeds removed
1 can (15 oz) kidney beans, drained and rinsed
1 cup cooked brown rice
1 cup diced tomatoes
1/2 cup diced onions
1/2 cup diced bell peppers
1 teaspoon chili powder
1/2 teaspoon cumin
Salt and pepper to taste
1 cup shredded cheese (optional)

Directions:

Preheat the oven to 375°F (190°C).
In a bowl, mix kidney beans, cooked brown rice, diced tomatoes, onions, bell peppers, chilli powder, cumin, salt, and pepper.
Fill each bell pepper half with the bean and rice mixture.

Place stuffed peppers in a baking dish and cover with foil.

Bake for 25-30 minutes until peppers are tender.If desired, sprinkle shredded cheese over the stuffed peppers during the last 5 minutes of baking.

Serving Size: Makes approximately 4 servings (1 stuffed pepper half per serving).Calories (per serving, without cheese): Approximately 200 calories.

20. Bean and Sweet Potato Hash:

Ingredients:

1 can (15 oz) black beans, drained and rinsed
2 medium sweet potatoes, peeled and diced
1 red bell pepper, diced
1 yellow onion, diced
2 cloves garlic, minced
1 teaspoon smoked paprika
1/2 teaspoon cumin
Salt and pepper to taste
2 tablespoons olive oil

Directions:

Heat olive oil in a large skillet over medium heat.
Add diced sweet potatoes and cook for 5-7 minutes until slightly softened.
Add diced onions and red bell pepper to the skillet.
Cook until vegetables are tender.
Stir in minced garlic, smoked paprika, cumin, salt, and pepper.
Add black beans to the skillet and cook for an additional 2-3 minutes until heated through.
Serve hot as a breakfast hash or a hearty side dish.
Serving Size: Makes approximately 4 servings.Calories (per serving): Approximately 250 calories.

58

Chapter 5

The Science Behind the Beans Diet

We delve into the scientific rationale behind the Beans Diet and explore how beans contribute to weight loss and overall health. Understanding the physiological mechanisms and research supporting the Beans Diet will provide you with the knowledge and confidence to embrace this dietary approach for long-term success.

Beans and Weight Loss:

The Beans Diet promotes weight loss through various mechanisms that harness the nutritional power of beans. One of the key factors is the high protein content found in beans. Protein plays a crucial role in weight management by increasing feelings of fullness, reducing appetite, and supporting muscle growth and repair. By incorporating beans into your meals, you can boost your protein intake and promote satiety, leading to reduced calorie consumption and improved weight loss outcomes.Furthermore, beans are rich in dietary fiber, which is essential for digestive health and weight management. Fiber adds bulk to the stool, promoting regular bowel movements and preventing constipation. Additionally, fiber slows down the digestion process, leading to a more gradual release of glucose into the bloodstream and improved blood sugar control. By keeping you feeling full for longer periods, fiber helps control hunger and reduce overall calorie intake, facilitating weight loss.Another key aspect of the Beans Diet is its emphasis on whole, nutrient-dense foods. Beans are packed with essential vitamins, minerals, and antioxidants that support overall health and well-being. By prioritising nutrient-rich foods like beans, you can ensure that your body receives the essential nutrients it needs to function optimally while promoting weight loss and reducing the risk of chronic diseases.Research Supporting the Beans Diet:Numerous studies have investigated the role of beans in weight management and overall health, providing robust scientific evidence supporting the Beans Diet. A systematic review and meta-analysis published in the American Journal of Clinical Nutrition found that diets rich in legumes, including beans, were associated with significantly lower body weight, body mass index (BMI), and waist circumference compared to diets low in legumes.Furthermore, a randomised controlled trial published in the Journal of the American College of Nutrition compared the effects of a bean-rich diet to a low-fat diet on weight loss and metabolic parameters in overweight and obese individuals. The study found that participants following the bean-rich diet experienced greater reductions in body weight, BMI, and waist circumference, as well as improvements in blood sugar levels and cholesterol levels, compared to those following the low-fat diet.Additionally, beans have been shown to have beneficial effects on appetite regulation and food intake. A study published in the journal Nutrients investigated the effects of white beans on appetite and satiety in overweight and obese individuals. The researchers found that consuming white beans as part of a meal resulted in increased feelings of fullness and reduced hunger compared to a meal without beans, suggesting that beans may help control appetite and reduce overall calorie intake.Overall, the scientific evidence supporting the Beans Diet is compelling, highlighting the potential of beans to promote weight loss, improve metabolic health, and support overall well-being. By incorporating beans into your diet and following the principles of the Beans Diet, you can harness the nutritional power of beans to achieve your weight loss goals and optimise your health.

Practical Tips for Success on the Beans Diet:

To maximise the benefits of the Beans Diet and achieve long-term success, it's essential to adopt healthy eating habits and lifestyle practices that support your weight loss goals. Here are some practical tips for success on the Beans Diet:

Prioritise Whole, Nutrient-Dense Foods: Focus on incorporating whole, nutrient-dense foods like beans, fruits, vegetables, whole grains, nuts, and seeds into your meals. These foods provide essential vitamins, minerals, and antioxidants that support overall health and well-being while promoting weight loss.

Practice Portion Control: Be mindful of portion sizes and avoid overeating, even when consuming healthy foods like beans. Use smaller plates, bowls, and utensils to help control portion sizes and listen to your body's hunger and fullness cues.

Cook Beans from Scratch: While canned beans are convenient and used in recipes in this book, cooking beans from scratch allows you to control the sodium content and seasoning of your beans. Soak dried beans overnight and cook them with herbs and spices for added flavour without relying on excessive salt or unhealthy fats.

Experiment with Different Bean Varieties: Explore the wide variety of beans available, including black beans, chickpeas, lentils, kidney beans, and more. Experiment with different bean varieties and recipes to keep your meals exciting and satisfying on your Beans Diet journey.

Stay Hydrated: Drink plenty of water throughout the day to stay hydrated and support optimal digestion. Aim to drink at least eight glasses of water per day, and consider incorporating hydrating foods like fruits and vegetables into your meals and snacks.

Be Active: In addition to following a healthy diet, incorporate regular physical activity into your routine to support weight loss and overall health. Aim for at least 150 minutes of moderate-intensity exercise or 75 minutes of vigorous-intensity exercise per week, as recommended by the Centers for Disease Control and Prevention (CDC).

Practise Mindful Eating: Pay attention to your eating habits and practise mindful eating by chewing your food slowly, savouring each bite, and avoiding distractions like television or smartphones while eating. This can help you enjoy your meals more fully and prevent overeating.

Chapter 6:

Overcoming Challenges and Staying Motivated on the Beans Diet

Embarking on any dietary journey, including the Beans Diet, can present its own set of challenges. In Chapter 6, we will explore common obstacles faced by individuals following the Beans Diet and provide practical strategies to overcome these challenges. Additionally, we will discuss effective methods for staying motivated and maintaining long-term success on the Beans Diet.

Common Challenges on the Beans Diet:

Limited Variety:

While beans are incredibly versatile, some individuals may find it challenging to incorporate them into their meals in creative and varied ways. Eating the same bean-based dishes repeatedly can lead to boredom and dissatisfaction with the diet.Digestive Issues: For some people, consuming beans can lead to digestive discomfort, such as bloating, gas, or stomach upset. This may be due to the high fiber content found in beans, which some individuals may have difficulty digesting.

Social Pressures:

Following a specific dietary plan like the Beans Diet may sometimes lead to social pressures or challenges, especially when dining out or attending social gatherings where bean-based options may be limited.

Cravings and Temptations:

Cravings for unhealthy foods or temptations to stray from the Beans Diet may arise, particularly during moments of stress, emotional upheaval, or exposure to enticing food advertisements.

Strategies to Overcome Challenges:

Experiment with Recipes: To combat limited variety, explore new recipes and cooking methods to keep your meals exciting and enjoyable. Look for creative bean-based dishes from various cuisines around the world and incorporate them into your meal rotation.Gradually Increase Fiber Intake: If you experience digestive issues when consuming beans, gradually increase your fiber intake over time to allow your body to adjust. Start with smaller portions of beans and gradually increase the serving size as your tolerance improves.

Additionally, soak dried beans before cooking and incorporate other fiber-rich foods like fruits, vegetables, and whole grains into your diet to support digestive health.

Plan Ahead for Social Situations: Before attending social gatherings or dining out, plan ahead by checking the menu for bean-based options or bringing a bean-based dish to share. Communicate your dietary preferences to friends and family members in advance to ensure that they can accommodate your needs.

Practise Mindful Eating: When faced with cravings or temptations, practise mindful eating by tuning into your body's hunger and fullness cues. Ask yourself if you are truly hungry or if you are eating out of boredom, stress, or habit. Find alternative ways to address emotional needs or cravings, such as going for a walk, practising relaxation techniques, or engaging in a hobby.

Staying Motivated on the Beans Diet:Set Realistic Goals:

Set realistic and achievable goals for yourself on the Beans Diet, taking into account your personal preferences, lifestyle, and health status. Break down larger goals into smaller, manageable steps and celebrate your progress along the way.

Track Your Progress: Keep track of your dietary habits, weight loss progress, and other relevant metrics using a food journal, mobile app, or other tracking tools. Monitoring your progress can help you stay accountable and motivated on your journey.

Find Support: Seek support from friends, family members, or online communities who share similar dietary goals and experiences. Having a support network can provide encouragement, accountability, and motivation during challenging times.

Focus on Non-Scale Victories: Instead of solely focusing on the number on the scale, celebrate non-scale victories such as increased energy levels, improved mood, better sleep, and enhanced overall well-being. These indicators of progress can be just as meaningful and motivating as weight loss itself.

Practice Self-Compassion: Be kind to yourself and practice self-compassion on your Beans Diet journey. Accept that setbacks and challenges are a natural part of the process and treat yourself with kindness and understanding during difficult times. Remember that every step forward, no matter how small, is progress towards your goals.

Reward Yourself: Reward yourself for reaching milestones and achieving your goals on the Beans Diet. Treat yourself to non-food rewards such as a relaxing bath, a new book, or a day trip to your favourite destination as a way to celebrate your accomplishments and stay motivated.

Stay Flexible: Be flexible and open-minded in your approach to the Beans Diet, recognizing that dietary preferences and needs may change over time. Allow yourself to experiment with different foods, recipes, and meal plans to find what works best for you and fits into your lifestyle.

Chapter 7:

Sustainable Lifestyle Changes for Long-Term Success

Our focus here is on the importance of sustainable lifestyle changes for achieving long-term success on the Beans Diet. While short-term diets may yield quick results, they often fail to provide lasting benefits. The Beans Diet emphasises the adoption of sustainable habits that promote overall health and well-being, ensuring that you not only lose weight but also maintain your results over time.

The Importance of Sustainability:

Sustainability is a key principle of the Beans Diet, emphasising the importance of making dietary and lifestyle changes that are realistic, enjoyable, and maintainable in the long run. Unlike fad diets that promote extreme restrictions or temporary fixes, the Beans Diet encourages gradual, sustainable changes that become integrated into your daily routine and support lifelong health and wellness.By focusing on sustainability, you can avoid the pitfalls of yo-yo dieting and weight cycling, which can have negative effects on metabolism, body composition, and overall health. Sustainable lifestyle changes promote consistency, balance, and flexibility, allowing you to maintain your progress and achieve lasting results on the Beans Diet.

Balanced Nutrition:

Focus on balanced nutrition by incorporating a variety of nutrient-dense foods into your diet, including beans, fruits, vegetables, whole grains, lean proteins, and healthy fats. Aim for a balanced plate at each meal, with a combination of carbohydrates, protein, and healthy fats to support energy levels, satiety, and overall health.

Regular Physical Activity: Make regular physical activity a priority in your daily routine to support weight management, improve cardiovascular health, and enhance overall well-being. Find activities that you enjoy and make them a regular part of your lifestyle, whether it's walking, jogging, cycling or swimming.

Adequate Sleep: Prioritise adequate sleep by aiming for 7-9 hours of quality sleep per night. Quality sleep is essential for overall health and well-being, supporting metabolism, hormone regulation, cognitive function, and mood. Create a relaxing bedtime routine and establish a consistent sleep schedule to optimise sleep quality.

Stress Management: Manage stress through effective coping strategies such as meditation, deep breathing exercises, yoga, journaling, or spending time in nature. Chronic stress can negatively impact health and contribute to weight gain, so it's important to find healthy ways to manage stress and promote relaxation.

Social Support: Surround yourself with a supportive network of friends, family members, or online communities who share similar health and wellness goals. Social support can provide encouragement, accountability, and motivation during challenging times, making it easier to stay on track with your goals.

Self-Care: Prioritise self-care by engaging in activities that promote relaxation, rejuvenation, and self-reflection. Take time for yourself each day to recharge and nurture your physical, emotional, and mental well-being. Whether it's reading a book, taking a bath, practising mindfulness, or pursuing a hobby, self-care is essential for maintaining balance and resilience.

Maintaining Long-Term Success:

Focus on Progress, Not Perfection: Shift your mindset from perfectionism to progress by celebrating small victories and focusing on the positive changes you've made. Recognize that setbacks are a natural part of the journey and use them as learning opportunities to adjust and continue moving forward.

Set Realistic Expectations: Set realistic and achievable goals for yourself, taking into account your personal preferences, lifestyle, and health status. Break down larger goals into smaller, manageable steps and celebrate your progress along the way.

Practice Consistency: Consistency is key to long-term success on the Beans Diet. Make healthy eating and lifestyle habits a consistent part of your daily routine, even on weekends or during holidays. Consistency builds momentum and helps reinforce positive habits over time.Stay Flexible: Be flexible and adaptable in your approach to the Beans Diet, recognizing that life is dynamic and circumstances may change. Allow yourself to enjoy occasional treats or deviations from your usual routine without guilt, and focus on getting back on track rather than dwelling on setbacks.

Reflect and Adjust: Regularly assess your progress, challenges, and goals, and be willing to adjust your approach as needed. Reflect on what is working well for you and what could be improved, and make adjustments accordingly to support your long-term success.

Seek Support: Seek support from friends, family members, or health professionals who can provide encouragement, accountability, and guidance on your journey. Surround yourself with positive influences who support your health and wellness goals and can help you stay motivated during challenging times.

Practice Self-Compassion: Be kind to yourself and practice self-compassion on your Beans Diet journey. Accept that progress may not always be linear, and setbacks are a natural part of the process. Treat yourself with kindness and understanding, and celebrate your efforts and achievements along the way.

Chapter 8

Maintaining Success and Embracing a Lifetime of Health

In Chapter 8, we shift our focus to the long-term maintenance of success achieved through the Beans Diet. While reaching your weight loss goals is an important milestone, maintaining those achievements and embracing a lifetime of health and wellness require ongoing dedication and commitment. This chapter explores strategies for sustaining your progress, navigating challenges, and cultivating a mindset that supports lifelong health.

Consistency is Key:

Consistency is crucial for maintaining success on the Beans Diet. Continue to prioritise balanced nutrition, regular physical activity, adequate sleep, stress management, and other healthy habits that have contributed to your success thus far.

Consistency reinforces positive behaviours and helps prevent relapses.

Set Realistic Expectations:

Maintain realistic expectations about your progress and embrace the concept of progress over perfection. Understand that maintaining weight loss and health improvements is a lifelong journey that may involve ups and downs. Celebrate your achievements and focus on continuous improvement rather than perfection.

Stay Accountable: Accountability is essential for long-term success. Stay accountable to yourself by tracking your dietary habits, physical activity, and other health behaviours. Consider joining a support group, working with a health coach, or enlisting the support of friends and family members who can help keep you motivated and accountable.

Adjust as Needed: Be flexible and willing to adjust your approach as needed to maintain your progress. Life circumstances, preferences, and goals may change over time, so it's important to adapt your dietary and lifestyle habits accordingly. Regularly reassess your goals and make adjustments as necessary to stay on track.

Navigating Challenges:Anticipate Setbacks: Setbacks are a natural part of any journey, including weight loss and health improvement. Anticipate potential challenges and setbacks, such as holidays, vacations, or periods of increased stress, and develop strategies for overcoming them. Remember that setbacks are temporary and can be managed with resilience and determination.

Learn from Setbacks: View setbacks as learning opportunities rather than failures. Reflect on the factors that contributed to the setback and identify actionable steps you can take to prevent similar challenges in the future. Use setbacks as opportunities for growth and self-improvement.

Practice Self-Compassion:

Be kind to yourself during difficult times and practice self-compassion. Recognize that setbacks are a normal part of the journey and treat yourself with understanding and forgiveness. Reframe negative self-talk into positive affirmations that reinforce your commitment to health and well-being.

Cultivating a Mindset for Lifelong Health:Embrace a Growth Mindset: Adopt a growth mindset, which focuses on continuous learning, improvement, and resilience. Embrace challenges as opportunities for growth, believe in your ability to change and adapt, and approach setbacks as temporary obstacles on the path to success.

Focus on Non-Scale Victories: Shift your focus away from the number on the scale and celebrate non-scale victories that reflect improvements in overall health and well-being. Celebrate achievements such such as increased energy levels, improved mood, better sleep, enhanced fitness levels, and positive changes in body composition.

Find Joy in Healthy Living: Cultivate a sense of joy and fulfilment in healthy living. Focus on the positive aspects of nourishing your body with wholesome foods, engaging in physical activity, managing stress, and prioritising self-care. Find activities and habits that bring you joy and make them a regular part of your routine.

Practice Gratitude: Cultivate an attitude of gratitude for your health and well-being. Take time each day to reflect on the things you are grateful for, including the progress you've made on your health journey.

Practising gratitude can help shift your mindset towards positivity and resilience, even during challenging times.Set New Goals: Continuously challenge yourself to set new goals and pursue new opportunities for growth and self-improvement. Whether it's trying new recipes, exploring different forms of physical activity, or engaging in personal development activities, setting new goals can keep you motivated and engaged in your health journey.

Chapter 9

Conclusion:

In conclusion, the Beans Diet offers a sustainable and enjoyable approach to weight loss and overall health. By harnessing the nutritional power of beans and embracing healthy lifestyle habits, you can achieve your health and wellness goals while enjoying delicious and nutritious meals. As you continue on your journey with the Beans Diet, remember to stay committed, stay resilient, and stay inspired to live your best life. Here's to a lifetime of health and happiness with the Beans Diet!

Printed in Great Britain
by Amazon